Getting Ready for My Tonsil Surgery

Tonsils Book for Kids – Preparation and Recovery

This book belongs to:

_____

Written by Dr. Fei Zheng-Ward   Illustrated by Moch. Fajar Shobaru

Copyright © 2024 Fei Zheng-Ward

Identifiers: ISBN 979-8-89318-027-5 (eBook)
ISBN 979-8-89318-026-8 (paperback)

Did you know you can see your tonsils?

If you open your mouth **wide** and look in the mirror, you will likely see them in the back of your throat.

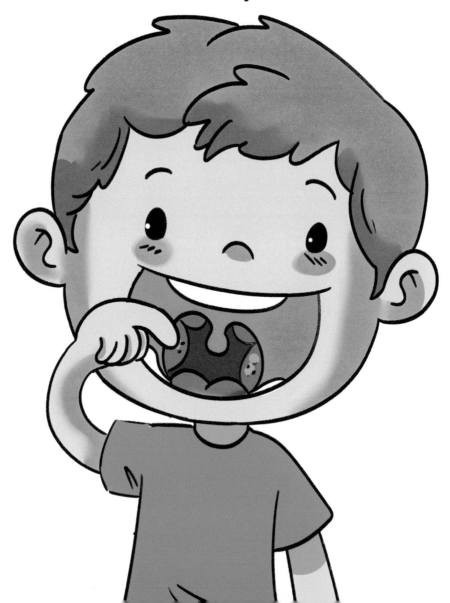

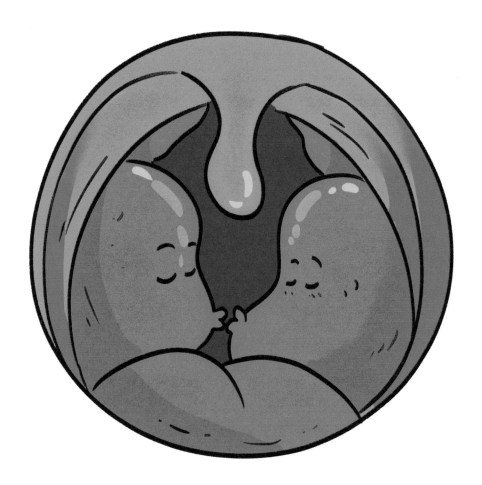

__*Fun fact*__: Kissing tonsils are **giant** tonsils that touch in the middle of the throat.

Do you have kissing tonsils?

____ YES ____ NO

Do you know what tonsils are?

They are one of many parts of your immune system that trap and fight germs to keep you healthy and strong.

Because your body has many *other* immune system parts, you don't have to have your tonsils, especially if they are making you feel unwell.

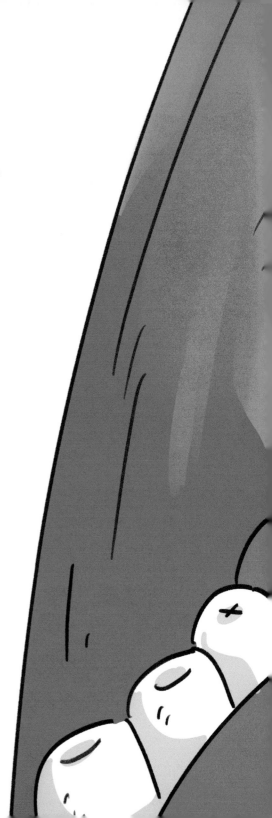

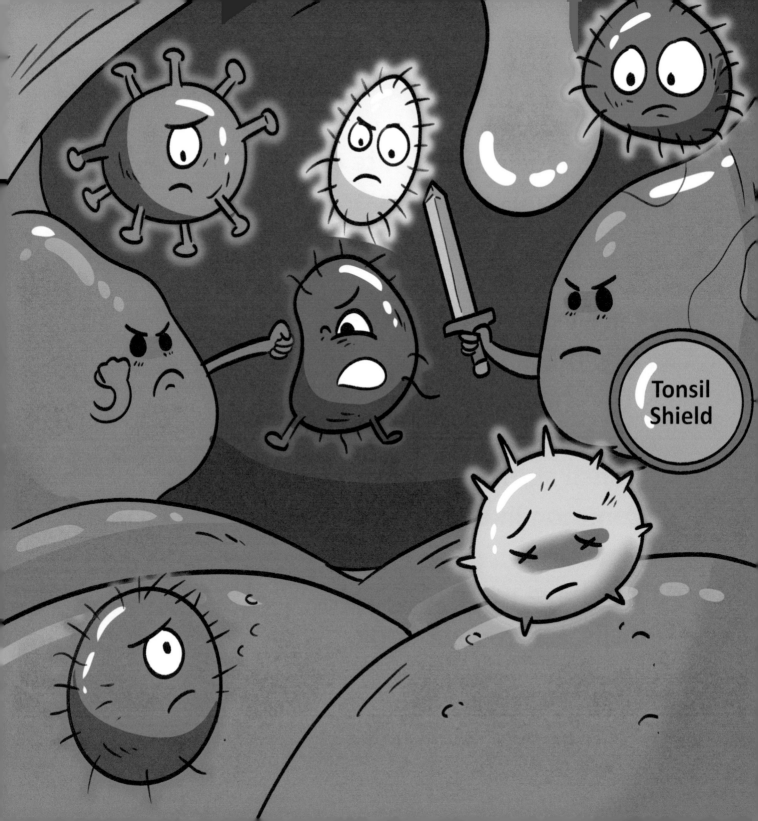

Interesting fact: Tiny white or yellow stones can form on your tonsils.

They are called tonsil stones. Usually, these stones will not harm you.

Tonsil stones are not common in children.

If you have them on your tonsils, take a good look.

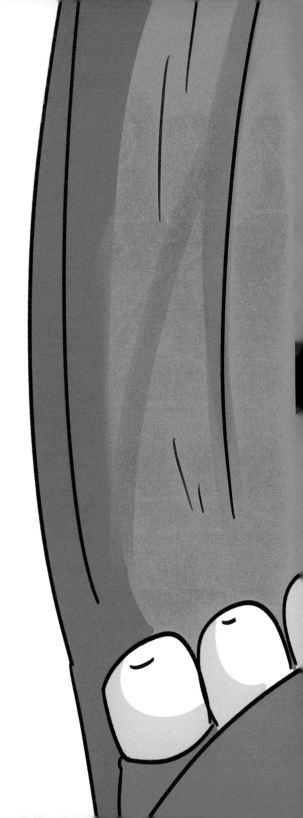

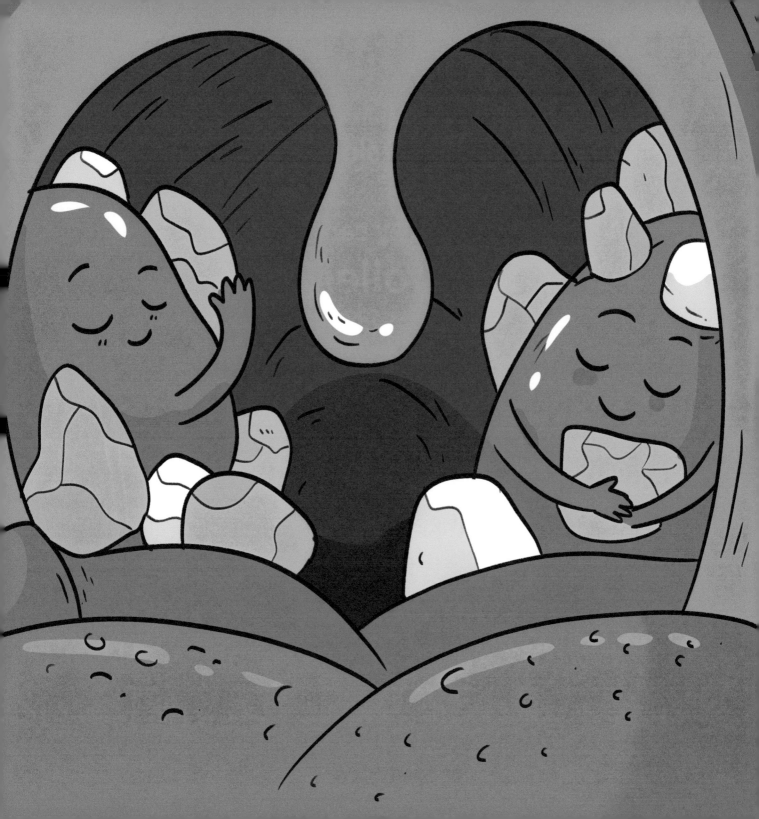

Your tonsils can get sick, too.

When they do, they can get
red and **swollen**.

Usually, they get better on their own.

When they don't, your doctor may
give you some medicine to take to
help them get better.

Sometimes, they keep getting sick,
which can make you sick as well.

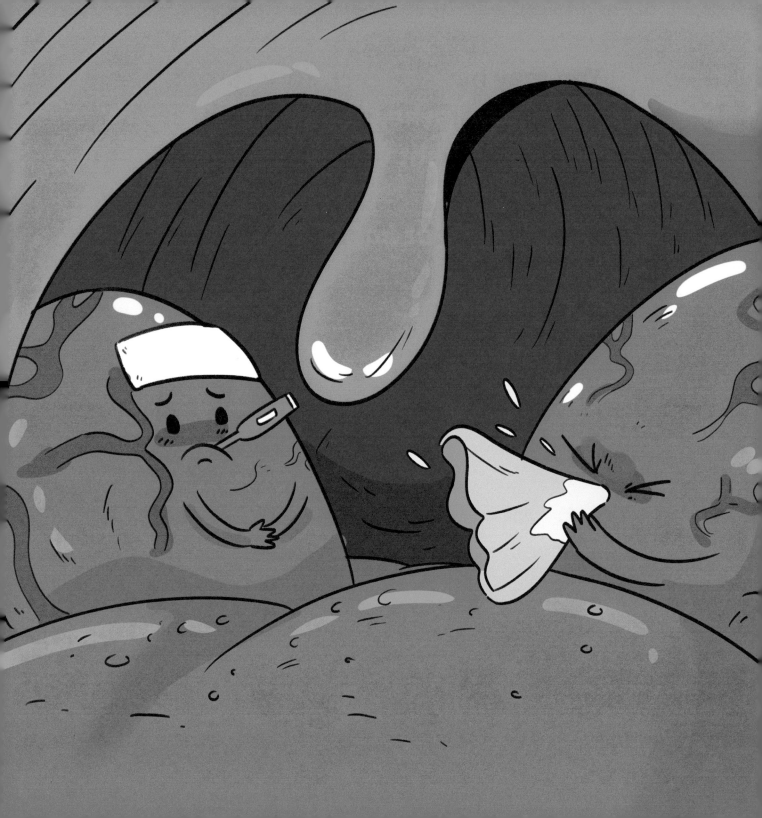

You may have a fever, sore throat, headache, earache, stinky breath, and don't want to eat much.

Has any of that happened to you?

_____ YES   _____ NO

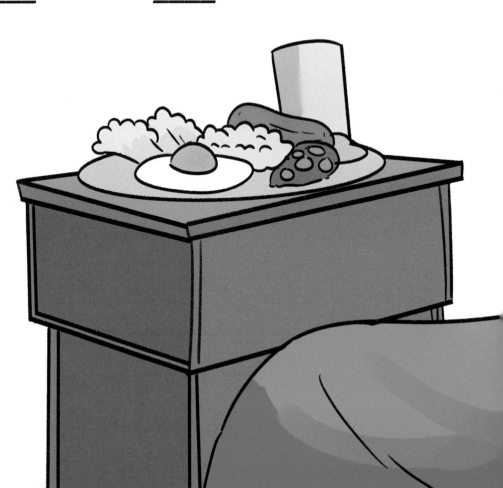

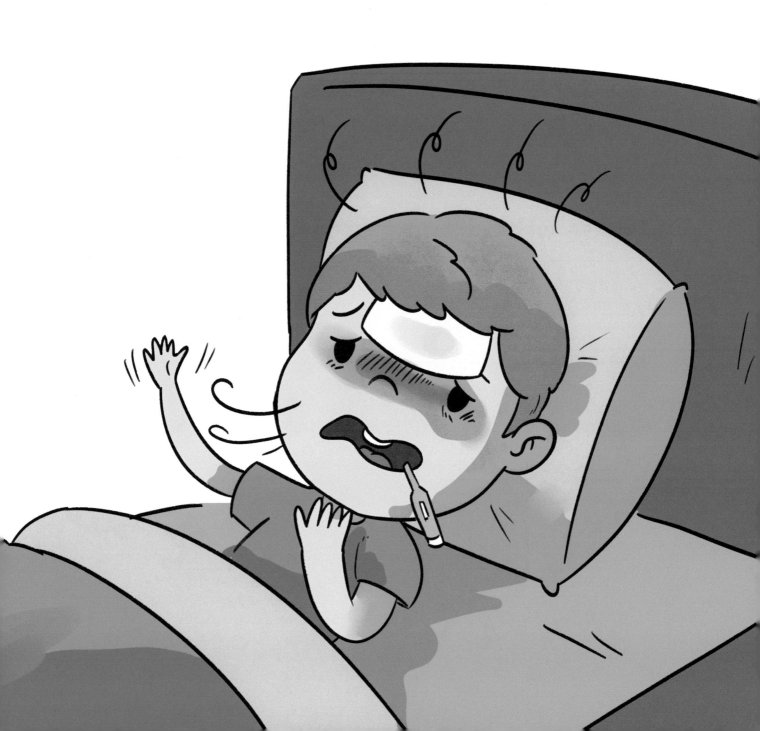

It can be difficult eating and swallowing when your throat hurts.

But try to drink water, juice, or your favorite drink to help your body fight the germs and get better.

Please write down your favorite drink below.

_____

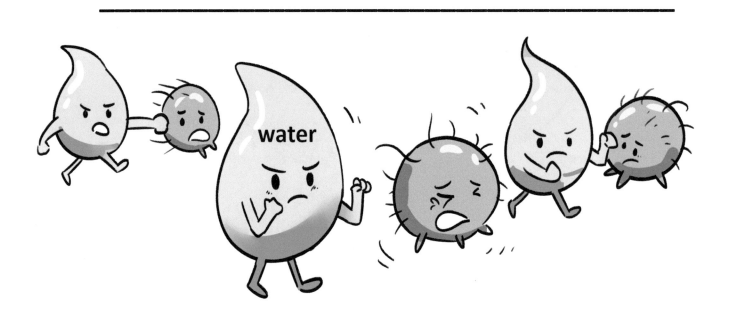

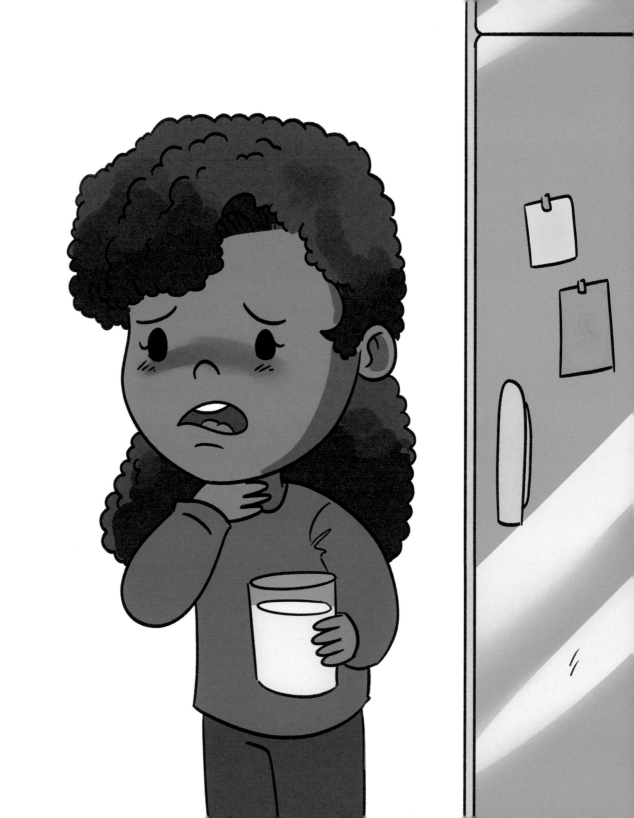

Sometimes, your swollen tonsils can make you snore loudly like a bear.

Did anyone tell you you snore at night?

_____ YES   _____ NO

What animal do you think snores the loudest?

Please write your answer below.

_____

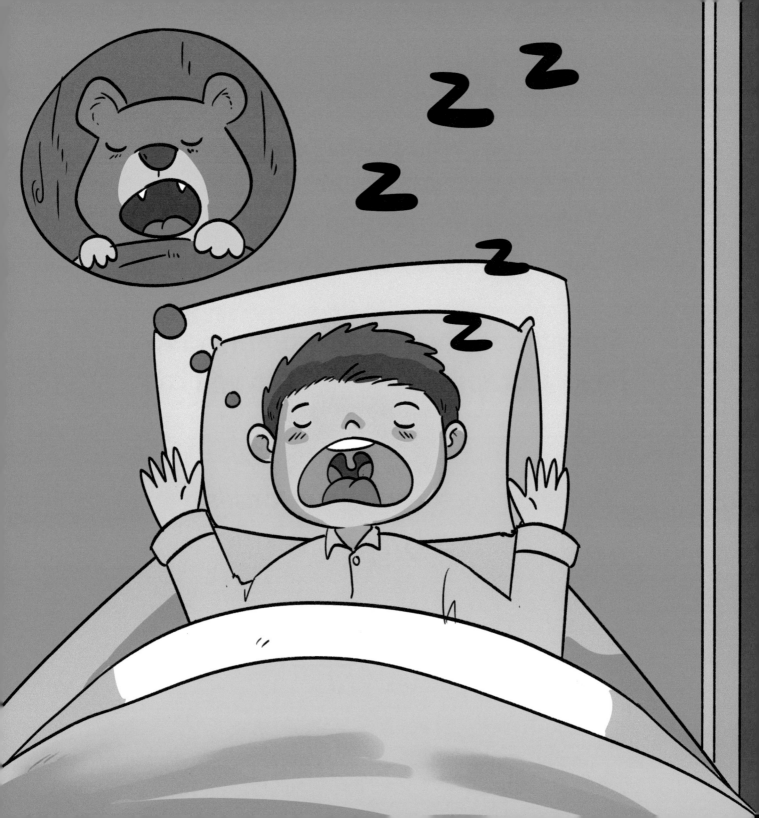

Your doctor, who is caring and gentle, can listen to your heart and lungs, check your ears and nose, and examine your tonsils.

Sometimes, they may recommend to have your tonsils removed so you can feel better.

Did your doctor say your tonsils are
big?

_____ YES   _____ NO

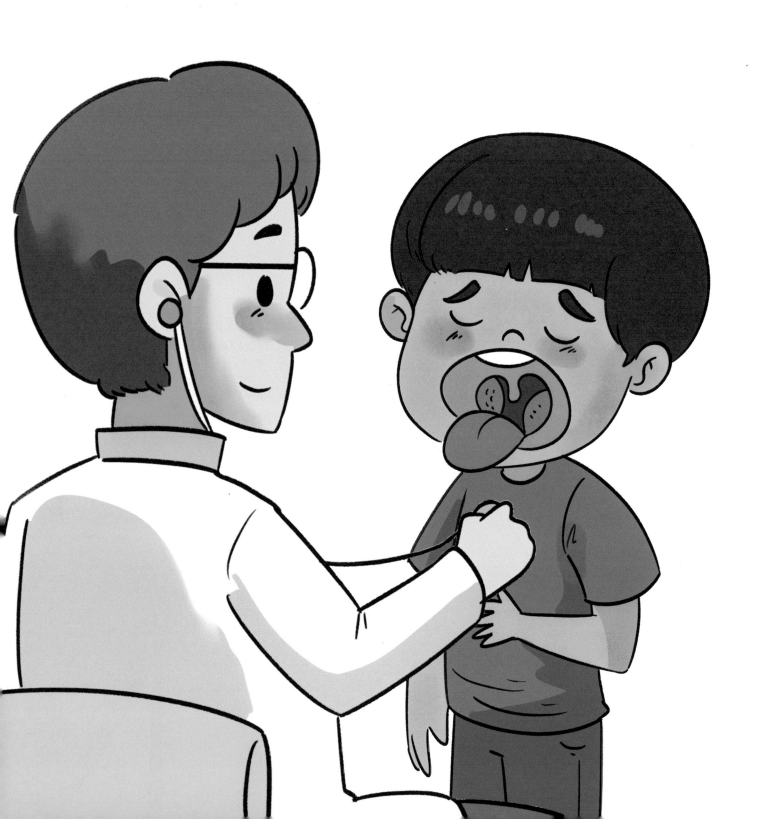

Your friendly doctor can easily remove your tonsils. It is a quick and simple surgery, and you won't feel a thing!

You will be sleeping and dreaming away while the surgery is underway.

What do you want to dream about during your surgery?

Your tonsils will be all gone before you wake up from your surgery.

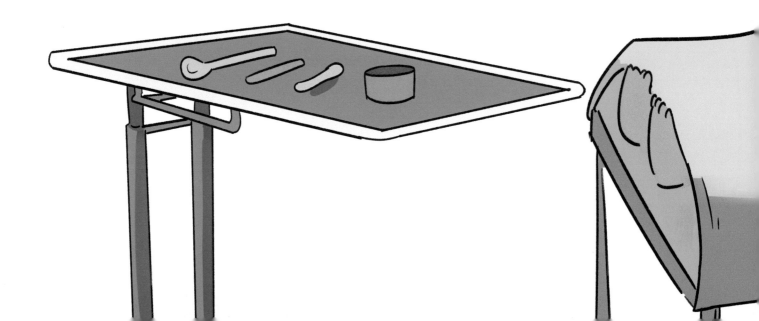

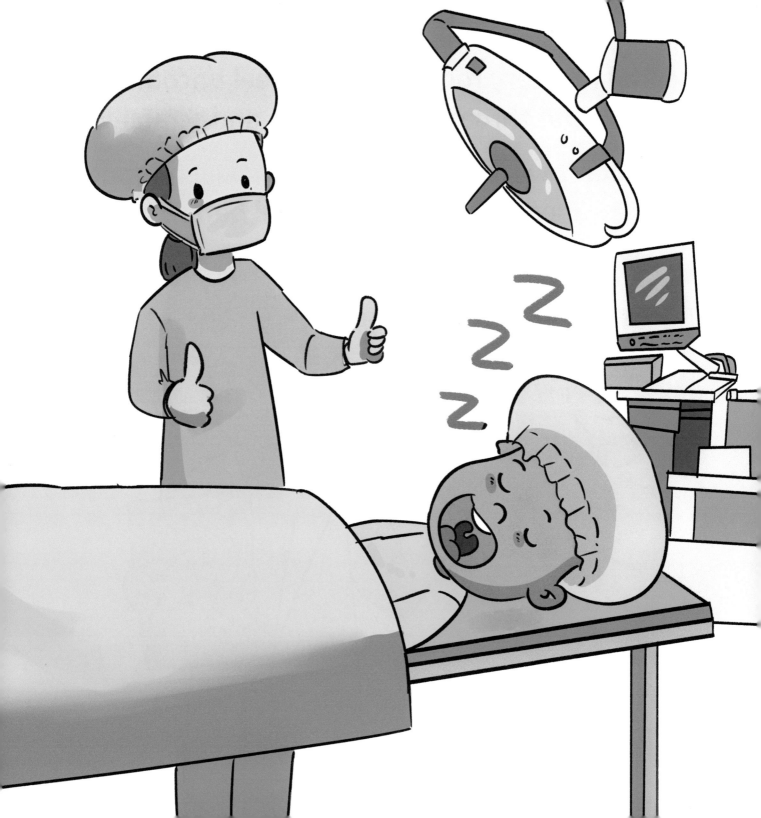

After your surgery is done, you will wake up in the hospital recovery room. You may feel uncomfortable, and your throat may feel sore and scratchy.

But don't worry, your nurse will give you special medicine to help you feel better.

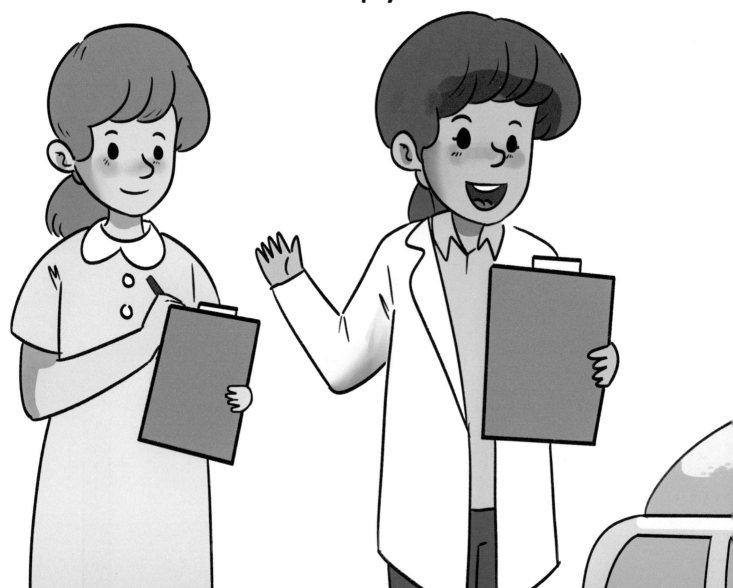

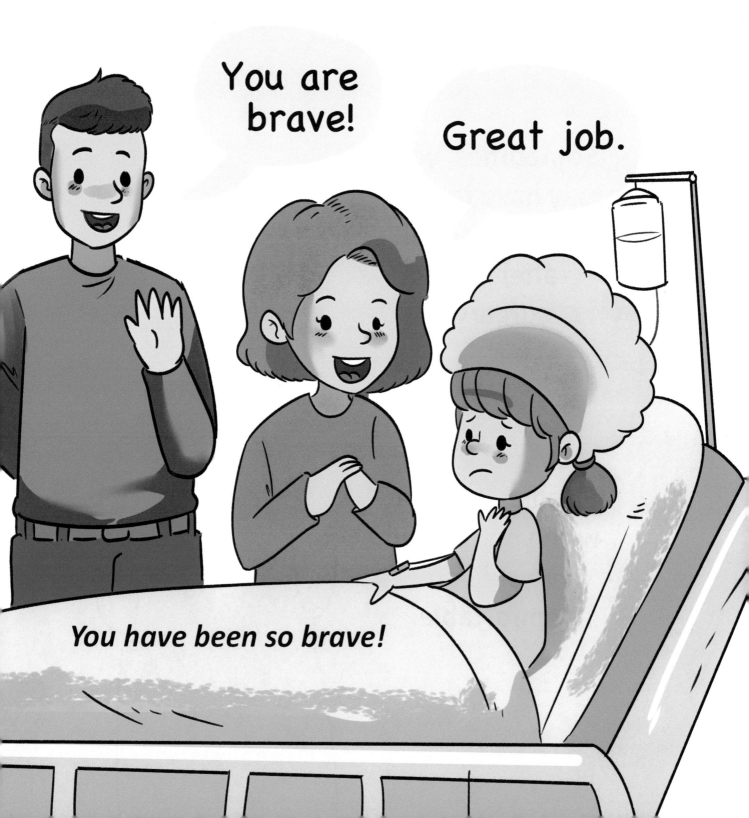

Sometimes, you may have to stay in the hospital after your surgery.

Your parent or guardian can stay with you to keep you safe and comfortable.

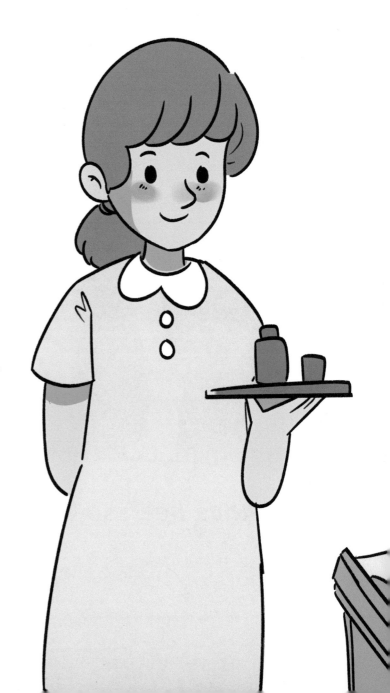

You can go home once you're feeling better.

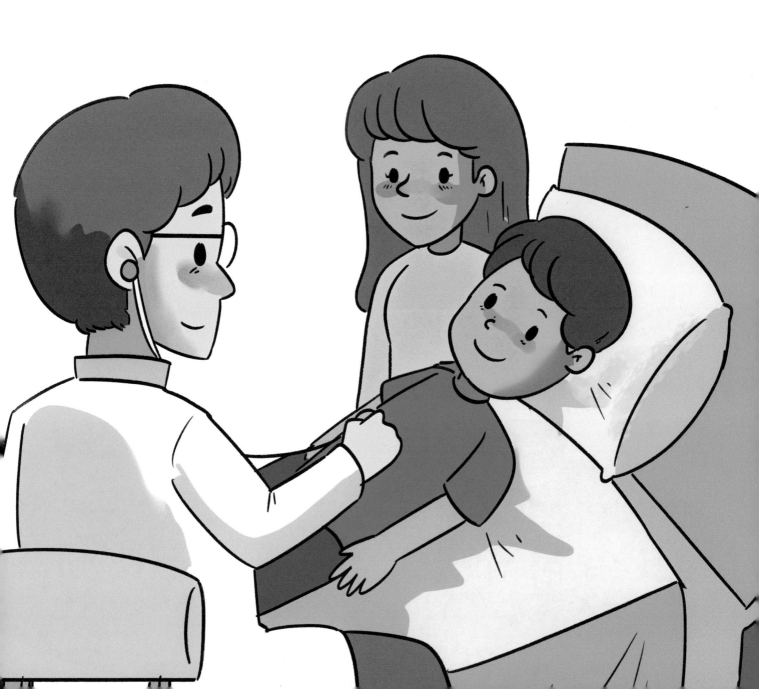

After your tonsils are removed, you will start feeling better soon.

But first, you get to eat ice cream or popsicles, and lots of them, too!

What is your favorite flavor?

_____

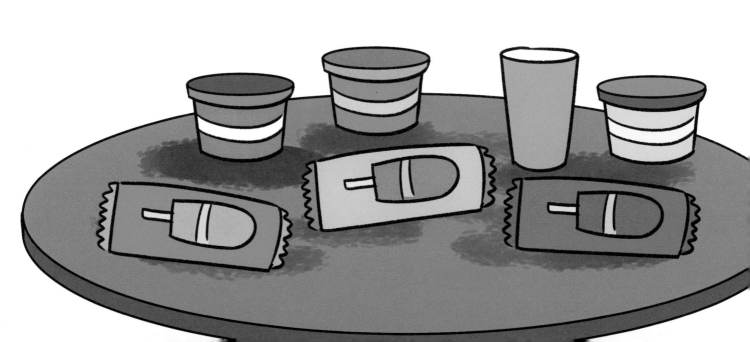

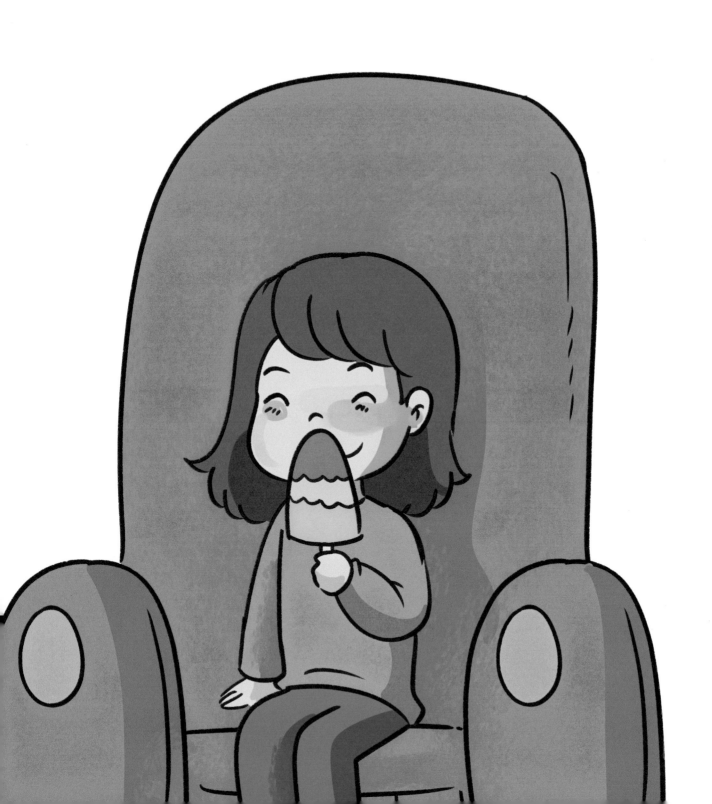

In addition to the ice cream and popsicles, please remember to drink water, juice, or your favorite drink or smoothie to help your body get better sooner.

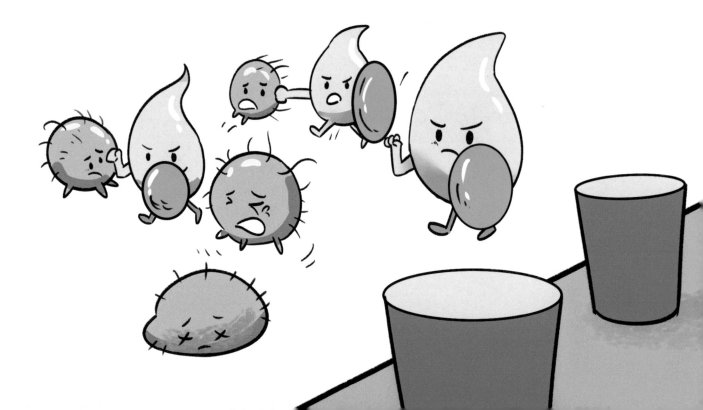

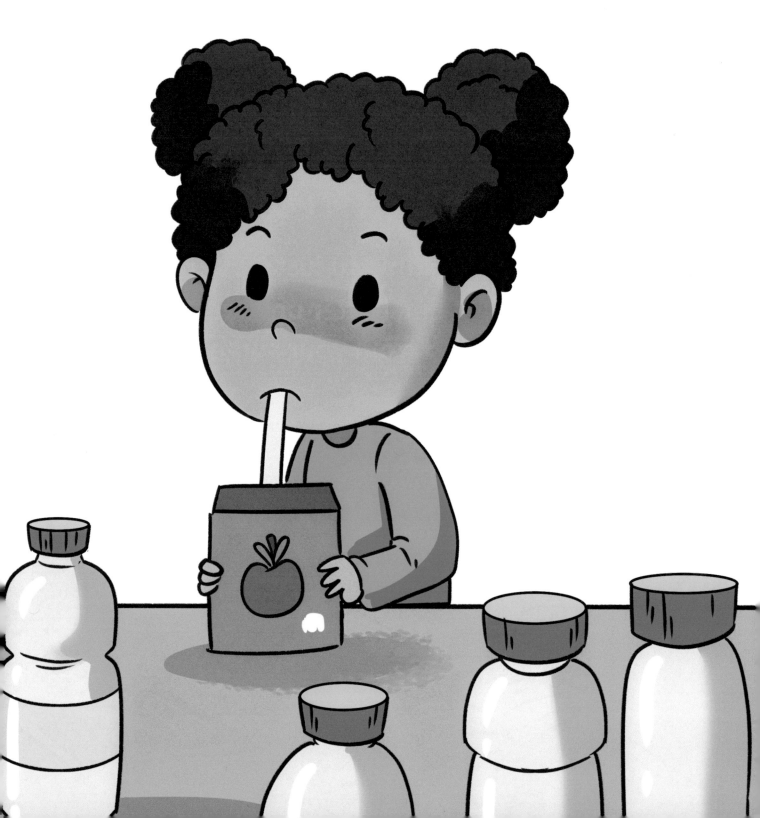

While you're recovering from your surgery, please take it easy.

You can read your favorite books, watch your favorite movies, or play card games.

This is a great time to just *relax* and focus on getting better until you have recovered from your surgery.

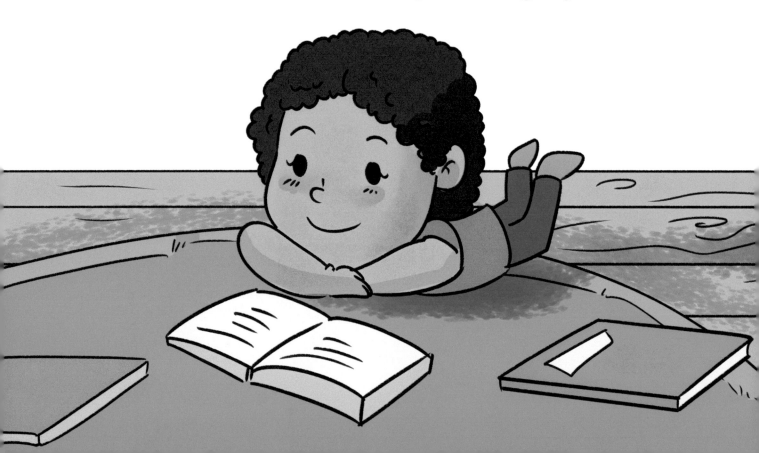

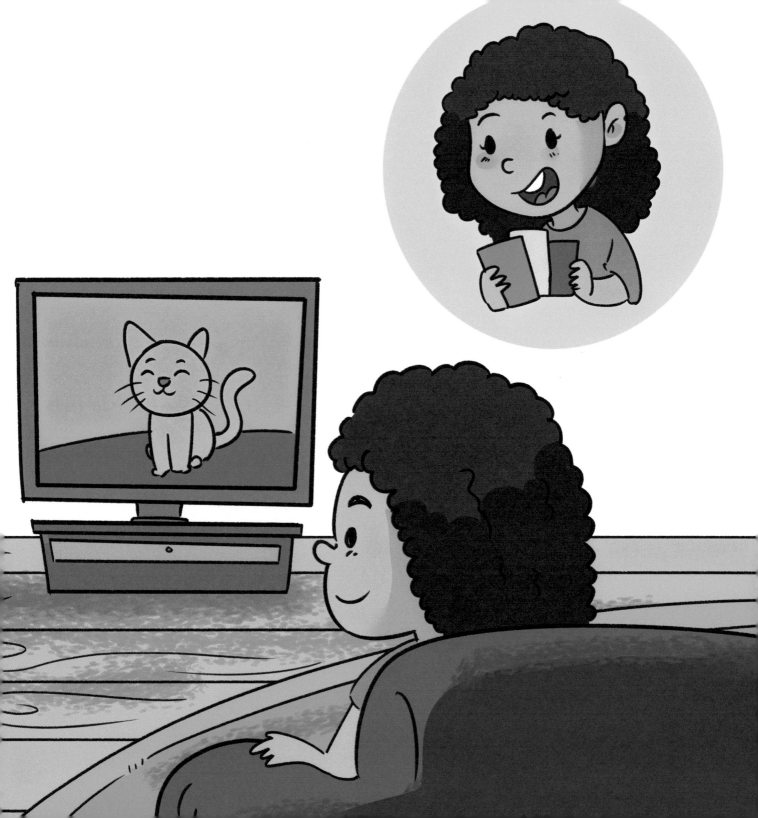

Soon, you will notice you can breathe and feel better, and your throat will not hurt like before.

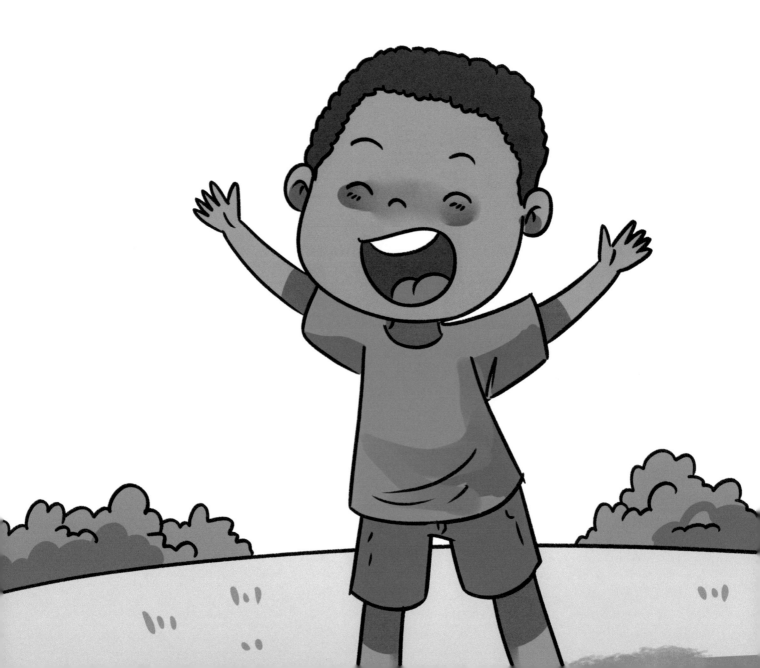

And you will sleep more comfortably (no more bear snores!).

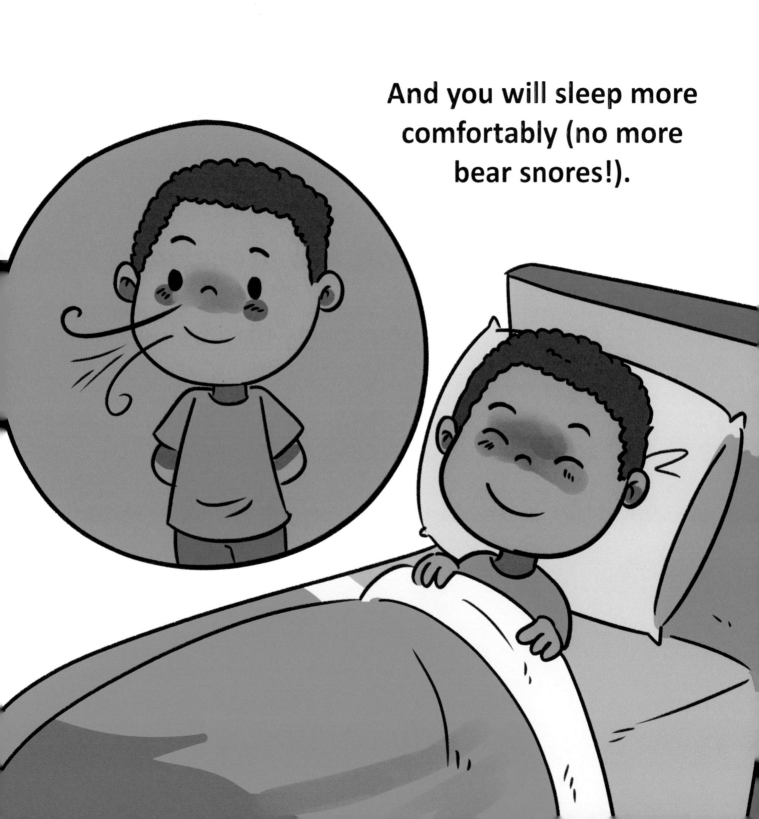

What will you do after your tonsils are gone?

A party? A celebration?

What's your favorite way to celebrate?

Draw or write your party plan below.

Speedy recovery!

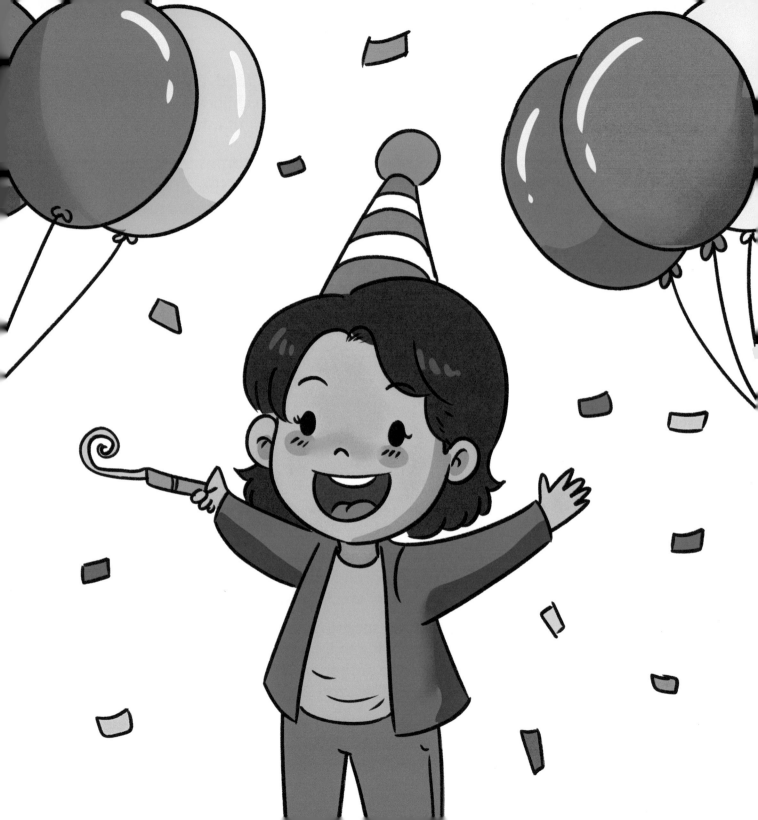

Notes for Parent/Guardian

*Tonsil stones are created because saliva, chewed-up food, and calcium surround the tonsils. These stones are rare in children.
Plus, they usually fall out on their own without intervention.

*After the surgery, it is common for children to feel confused, disoriented, or irritable, and they may cry, sob, kick, scream, or thrash around.
It normally takes about one hour for the anesthesia to wear off.

*Post-surgery instructions/restrictions:
Your child's doctor should give you specific instructions on (1) what your child can and cannot do during the recovery period, (2) the duration of the post-surgical restrictions, and (3) any post-surgical follow-ups. Additionally, (4) they should instruct what to watch out for and when it is necessary for you to bring your child back to the hospital in case of an emergency. If they forget, please kindly remind them and obtain these instructions/restrictions before leaving the hospital.

Disclaimer

Did this picture book help your child in some way?
If so, I would love to hear about it!

www.amazon.com/gp/product-review/B0D9LL1PZN

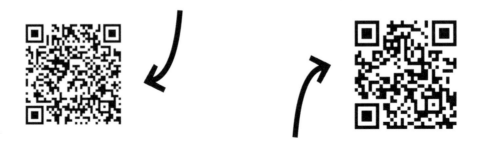

www.fzwbooks.com

Get 5 FREE coloring pages when you sign up for my email.

I would _love_ to see your child's beautiful artwork!

Please feel free to share their creative work to Instagram or Facebook.

Tag me (@FZWbooks) and use #FZWloveskids

Feel free to post any of these:

* Photos of them having fun coloring the free downloaded pages

* Photos of them reading or answering questions in this book

* Photos of them being brave and ready for their surgery

Instagram   Facebook

About the Author

Dr. Fei Zheng-Ward is a clinical anesthesiologist who understands the apprehension patients (both adults and children) may have surrounding their upcoming surgery. Her goal in her medical books is to bring useful information to patients so they have a better understanding and appreciation of what happens leading up to, during, and after surgery. She wants readers to be more empowered to make informed decisions and to feel more at ease with their surgery.

As a practicing physician, she takes pride in being respected for her attention to detail, commitment to providing compassionate and personalized patient care, and strong presence in patient advocacy in the perioperative period for each of her patients. She understands the importance of physical and emotional well-being and advocates for patient autonomy.

In addition to her clinical practice, Dr. Zheng-Ward is actively involved in medical education and contributes to medical journals and state and national conferences.

She is an award-winning author for her book titled *What to Expect and How to Prepare for Your Surgery.*

More about Dr. Fei Zheng-Ward:

* Board Certified Anesthesiologist

* Anesthesiology Residency Training at The Johns Hopkins Hospital in Baltimore, MD

* Master in Public Health (MPH) degree from Dartmouth Medical School in Hanover, NH

Books by the author

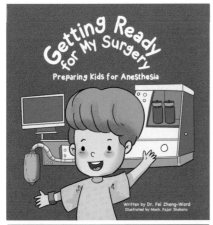

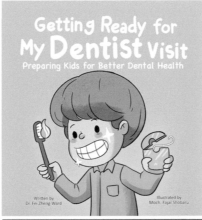

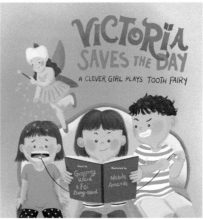

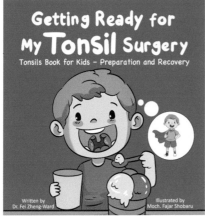

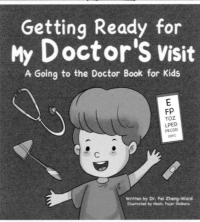

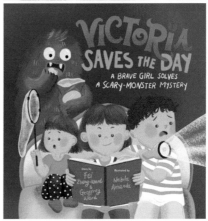

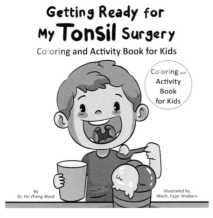

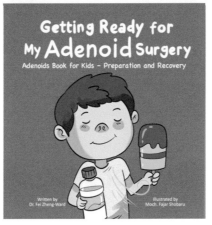

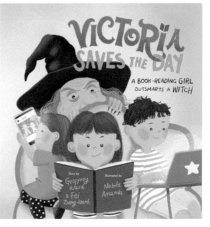

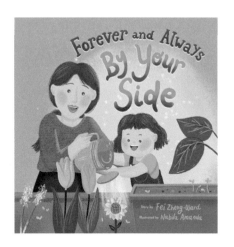

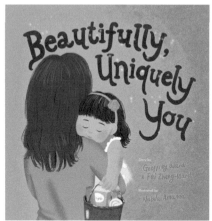

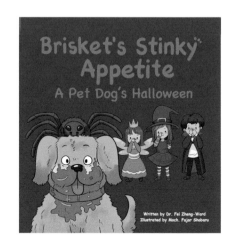

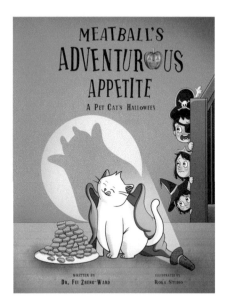

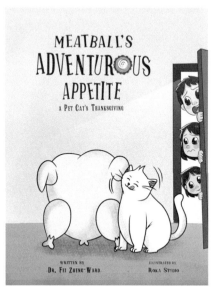

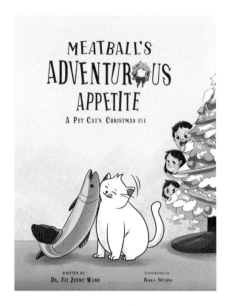

Follow the author for more upcoming titles.

Made in United States
Troutdale, OR
11/11/2024